MW00469235

THE COMPLETE GUIDE TO USE XENICAL

The Complete Guide on How to Treat Obesity and Help Weight Loss by Blocking and Preventing the Absorption of Fats by the Human Body

ISBN 978-1-312-40400-7
Varick Ken
Copyright@2023

TABLE OF CONTENT

CHAPTER 1

INTRODUCTION

The medication Xenical, alternatively referred to as Orlistat, is commonly prescribed for the purpose of managing weight in individuals who are classified as overweight or obese. Xenical, which was sanctioned by the Food and Drug Administration (FDA) in the year 1999, functions as a lipase inhibitor by diminishing the assimilation of dietary fats. The present study endeavors to provide a comprehensive exposition elucidating the mechanism of action of Xenical, its various applications, recommended dosage, plausible adverse effects, contraindications, and precautions, while also underscoring salient factors that patients should take into account.

Xenical operates through the inhibition of pancreatic and gastric lipases, which are enzymes that facilitate the breakdown of dietary fats into absorbable forms. The process of inhibition effectively hinders the absorption of approximately 30% of fats that are ingested, leading to their subsequent excretion through fecal matter. Xenical facilitates weight loss by diminishing the caloric consumption derived from dietary fats.

Xenical is primarily prescribed for the management of obesity, in conjunction with a calorie-restricted diet and routine physical activity. Individuals who have a body mass index (BMI) of 30 or greater, or those with a BMI of 27 or greater and co-occurring risk factors such as hypertension, diabetes, or dyslipidemia are advised to take certain measures.

The recommended dosage and administration of Xenical involves taking 120 mg orally, three times a day, either immediately before, during, or up to one hour after each primary meal that contains fat. In the event that a meal is not consumed or lacks fat content, it is advisable to exclude the dosage. The recommended usage of Xenical involves its combination with a nutritionally balanced and reduced-calorie diet that comprises around 30% of calories derived from fat.

The efficacy of Xenical in facilitating weight reduction has been established through clinical investigations. Studies have demonstrated that the utilization of Xenical in conjunction with a calorie-restricted diet results in more significant weight reduction in comparison to relying solely on dietary modifications. Furthermore, it has exhibited enhancements in diverse cardiometabolic risk indicators, including but not limited to blood pressure, lipid profiles, and glycemic regulation.

The medication Xenical is typically well-tolerated, but it has the potential to induce gastrointestinal side effects as a result of the expulsion of undigested fats. The observed adverse reactions comprise of oily spotting, flatus with discharge, oily or fatty stools, augmented frequency of bowel movements, and abdominal discomfort. The aforementioned effects are frequently of a mild and temporary nature, exhibiting a reduction in intensity with the continuation of treatment.

Xenical should not be administered to individuals suffering from chronic malabsorption syndrome or cholestasis due to the potential for exacerbation of these conditions. It is advisable to refrain from its use during the gestational and lactation periods. Individuals who exhibit a documented hypersensitivity to Xenical or any of its constituent elements are advised against the use of this medication.

Individuals who have a medical history of kidney stones, pancreatitis, or gallbladder disease are advised to exercise prudence when utilizing Xenical. It is advisable to utilize a multivitamin supplement that comprises of fat-soluble vitamins (namely, vitamins A, D, E, and K) to guarantee sufficient vitamin consumption, as the absorption of these vitamins may be hindered by Xenical. Maintaining adequate hydration is imperative during the administration of Xenical.

Xenical has the potential to interact with specific pharmaceuticals such as cyclosporine, which is administered to transplant recipients, levothyroxine, utilized for the treatment of hypothyroidism, and anticoagulants like warfarin. The aforementioned interactions may require modifications in dosage or vigilant observation of the patient's state.

The prolonged utilization and sustenance of weight loss is not the intended purpose of Xenical. The determination of treatment duration ought to be made by healthcare professionals, taking into account the specific needs of each patient. The maintenance of weight loss over an extended period is contingent upon the continuation of lifestyle adjustments such as the adoption of healthy dietary patterns, consistent engagement in physical exercise, and the implementation of behavioral modifications.

Prior to commencing Xenical treatment, it is recommended that patients seek consultation with healthcare providers, such as physicians or registered dietitians, to evaluate their eligibility for the medication. These experts are capable of offering individualized recommendations concerning the appropriate dosage, dietary adjustments, and exercise regimens that are customized to meet the unique requirements of each patient.

In conclusion, Xenical, also known as Orlistat, is a pharmacological agent frequently employed for the purpose of weight management in individuals who are overweight or obese. Xenical facilitates weight loss when used in conjunction with a calorie-restricted diet and physical activity by impeding the assimilation of ingested fats. Although typically well-tolerated, this substance has the potential to induce gastrointestinal adverse reactions. It is imperative to take into account the contraindications and precautions associated with a particular treatment, and it is recommended that patients seek advice from healthcare professionals to determine its suitable application. It is important to note that Xenical should be considered as a singular component within a comprehensive weight management strategy. The achievement of successful weight loss and maintenance necessitates the adoption of long-term lifestyle modifications.

CHAPTER 2

IMPORTANT USES OF XENICAL

Xenical is a pharmaceutical preparation comprising orlistat as the principal active constituent, which is predominantly employed for the purpose of weight control. The mechanism of action involves inhibition of the assimilation of ingested fat within the organism, thereby resulting in a decrease in caloric consumption and facilitation of weight reduction. This written discourse aims to provide a comprehensive analysis of the applications of Xenical, delving into its modes of operation, prescribed amount, probable adverse reactions, and its significance in the treatment of obesity and associated ailments.

The mechanism of action of Xenical involves the inhibition of the lipase enzyme, which plays a crucial role in the hydrolysis of dietary fats into absorbable molecules. Xenical functions by inhibiting the activity of a specific enzyme, thereby impeding the process of digestion and absorption of approximately 33% of the ingested dietary fat. Subsequently, unabsorbed lipids are eliminated through defecation, resulting in a decrease in total caloric consumption and consequent reduction in body weight.

The standard prescribed amount of Xenical is 120 mg, which should be ingested orally thrice a day along with every major meal that includes fat. It is noteworthy that the utilization of Xenical ought to be accompanied by a calorie-restricted diet that is abundant in fruits, vegetables, and whole grains. It is recommended to consume the medication within a time frame of one hour after a meal or up to an hour subsequent to the ingestion of food.

The main application of Xenical is to manage weight in individuals who suffer from obesity or overweight conditions. This product is deemed appropriate for individuals who have reached adulthood as well as adolescents who are 12 years of age or older. Xenical can be an effective component of a holistic weight loss regimen that encompasses dietary modifications and physical activity, facilitating the attainment and sustenance of a more optimal body mass. It is noteworthy that Xenical should not be regarded as a panacea for weight loss, but rather as a mechanism that, if employed judiciously, can facilitate a weight control regimen.

The treatment of obesity is a crucial matter as it is a persistent ailment marked by an overabundance of body fat, which is linked to a range of health hazards including hypertension, diabetes, heart disease, and specific forms of cancer. Xenical has been demonstrated to be a viable therapeutic alternative for individuals suffering from obesity, as it facilitates weight loss and has the potential to ameliorate specific health conditions associated with obesity. Studies have demonstrated that the utilization of Xenical for weight reduction purposes is associated with enhancements in blood pressure, cholesterol profiles, and glycemic regulation.

The management of Type 2 diabetes involves addressing the metabolic disorder that is marked by elevated blood glucose levels resulting from insulin resistance. The presence of obesity is a notable contributor to the likelihood of developing type 2 diabetes. Xenical has the potential to enhance insulin sensitivity and glycemic control in individuals diagnosed with type 2 diabetes by facilitating weight loss. It is noteworthy that Xenical ought to be incorporated as a component of a comprehensive diabetes management strategy, which encompasses dietary adjustments, physical activity, and other medically prescribed drugs.

Polycystic Ovary Syndrome (PCOS) is a medical condition characterized by hormonal imbalances that primarily affects women within the reproductive age range. The condition is distinguished by elevated levels of androgens, irregular patterns of menstruation, and the existence of cysts in the ovaries. The condition of Polycystic

Ovary Syndrome (PCOS) is frequently linked with obesity, which has the potential to worsen the symptoms. The utilization of Xenical in conjunction with lifestyle modifications has the potential to aid in weight management among women with PCOS, thereby enhancing hormonal balance, menstrual regularity, and fertility outcomes.

Non-alcoholic fatty liver disease (NAFLD) is a pathological state marked by the excessive deposition of lipids within the hepatic tissue, resulting in hepatic inflammation and injury. The condition of being obese represents a noteworthy risk factor for Non-Alcoholic Fatty Liver Disease (NAFLD). The utilization of Xenical for weight reduction purposes has been found to be effective in diminishing liver fat content and enhancing liver function among individuals diagnosed with non-alcoholic fatty liver disease (NAFLD). Similar to other medical conditions, the utilization of Xenical necessitates incorporation into a comprehensive treatment regimen, which encompasses dietary modifications and consistent physical activity.

maintenance is a crucial aspect of weight loss management.

Sustaining weight loss is a critical component for achieving enduring success in the management of obesity. The phenomenon of yo-yo dieting, characterized by a recurring pattern of weight loss and regain, is a common experience among individuals who have successfully lost weight. Xenical has been found to be effective in weight maintenance as it lowers the probability of weight regain following an initial weight reduction. Xenical functions by impeding the absorption of fat, thereby promoting adherence to dietary modifications and fostering the cultivation of more salubrious eating behaviors.

The administration of Xenical, like any other medication, is linked to potential side effects. Possible academic rewrite: The clinical manifestations may encompass gastrointestinal signs and symptoms, such as steatorrhea, diarrhea, bloating, colicky discomfort, and anal leakage of stool. The mild side effects frequently arise as a result of the transit of undigested fat through the gastrointestinal tract. Adhering to the prescribed dosage and dietary recommendations is crucial in order to mitigate the occurrence of these adverse effects.

In summary, Xenical is a pharmaceutical agent that serves multiple purposes in the management of body weight and the treatment of medical conditions associated with obesity. Xenical has the potential to facilitate weight loss, enhance glycemic control in individuals with type 2 diabetes, alleviate symptoms of polycystic ovary syndrome (PCOS), mitigate liver fat accumulation in non-alcoholic fatty liver disease (NAFLD), and assist in weight management by impeding the absorption of dietary fat. It is imperative to incorporate Xenical into a comprehensive weight loss regimen that encompasses dietary modifications, consistent physical activity, and diligent medical oversight in order to attain the most favorable outcomes. It is advisable to seek personalized advice and guidance from a healthcare professional concerning the utilization of Xenical or any other medication.

CHAPTER 3

SIDE REACTIONS OF XENICAL

Orlistat, commonly referred to as Xenical, is a pharmaceutical drug that requires a prescription and is utilized for the purpose of managing weight loss. This medication pertains to a category of pharmaceuticals known as lipase inhibitors, which function by impeding the assimilation of ingested lipids within the gastrointestinal tract. Although Xenical has been shown to be efficacious in facilitating weight loss, it is crucial to acknowledge its possible adverse effects and hazards. This article will provide a comprehensive analysis of the potential side effects and risks associated with the use of Xenical.

It is imperative to acknowledge that the utilization of Xenical necessitates the oversight of a healthcare practitioner and integration into a holistic weight reduction regimen, prior to delving into the particular hazards and adverse reactions. The intervention in question cannot be considered a self-sufficient remedy for reducing body weight and must be complemented by a well-rounded nutritional regimen, consistent physical activity, and modifications in behavior.

Xenical is frequently associated with gastrointestinal adverse events, which constitute one of the most prevalent side effects. Due to its mechanism of action that involves inhibiting the absorption of dietary fats, Xenical may elicit adverse effects such as oily stools, flatulence, increased frequency of bowel movements, and heightened urgency to defecate. The aforementioned effects manifest due to the passage of undigested fats through the gastrointestinal tract, ultimately resulting in their excretion through fecal matter. The management of these adverse effects can be achieved through adherence to a low-fat dietary regimen and reduction in the consumption of high-fat food items.

Xenical may induce steatorrhea and fecal incontinence, resulting in the presence of oily stains on clothing or in the commode. On occasion, individuals may encounter bowel incontinence, a condition characterized by the incapacity to regulate bowel movements. The aforementioned effects have the potential to cause social discomfort and adversely affect the individual's overall well-being.

The use of Xenical may lead to vitamin and nutrient deficiencies due to its interference with fat absorption, which can consequently affect the absorption of fat-soluble vitamins, including vitamins A, D, E, and K. Prolonged utilization of Xenical may elevate the likelihood of insufficiencies in vital vitamins that play a crucial role in diverse physiological processes. It is advisable to consume a multivitamin supplement comprising the aforementioned vitamins at a minimum interval of two hours prior to or subsequent to the administration of Xenical.

Instances of severe liver injury have been linked to Xenical, albeit infrequently, with liver and kidney problems being a potential outcome. Indications of hepatic dysfunction encompass jaundice, darkened urine, abdominal discomfort, and anorexia. In the event of the manifestation of any of these symptoms, it is imperative to promptly seek medical attention. Furthermore, it is advisable for individuals who have preexisting liver or kidney conditions to exercise caution when using Xenical and to undergo close monitoring by their healthcare provider.

Xenical may elicit allergic reactions in certain individuals, presenting as symptoms such as pruritus, urticaria, edema, vertigo, or dyspnea. In the event of any manifestation of an allergic reaction, it is imperative to promptly seek medical assistance.

Xenical has the potential to interact with specific pharmaceuticals, including cyclosporine, an immunosuppressant, and warfarin, a blood thinner, thereby impacting their efficacy. It is imperative to apprise the healthcare practitioner of all medications being ingested to avert possible drug interactions.

The administration of Xenical is contraindicated during pregnancy and lactation. The available literature on the impact of Xenical on pregnant or lactating females is restricted, and its safety profile in these cohorts remains undetermined.

Psychological effects may arise as a result of weight loss medications, including Xenical, although they are not directly caused by the medication itself. Individuals may encounter alterations in their emotional state, physical perception, or self-worth. It is imperative to consult with a healthcare practitioner to ensure adequate assistance and direction during the process of weight reduction.

It is imperative to comprehend that the aforementioned side effects and risks are not comprehensive, and personal encounters may differ.

Prior consultation with a healthcare practitioner is imperative prior to initiating the use of Xenical or any pharmacological agent intended for weight reduction purposes. The healthcare professionals have the ability to offer customized recommendations, oversee your advancement, and assist in the management of any potential adverse reactions.

To summarize, although Xenical has demonstrated efficacy as a weight loss supplement, it is crucial to acknowledge its possible adverse effects and hazards. When utilizing Xenical, it is important to take into account various factors such as gastrointestinal complications, vitamin deficiencies, liver and kidney impairments, allergic responses, drug interferences, and psychological impacts. When Xenical is administered under the guidance of a healthcare practitioner and in conjunction with a comprehensive weight loss regimen, it is possible to optimize the advantages of weight reduction while minimizing the associated hazards.

CHAPTER 4

ADMINISTRATION AND DOSAGE OF XENICAL

The objective of this chapter is to furnish a comprehensive exposition of the recommended dosage and administration protocols for Xenical. This will encompass an elucidation of its mechanism of action, indications, contraindications, dosage formulations, dosing regimen, and considerations pertaining to its administration.

Xenical operates through the mechanism of action of inhibiting lipase, thereby classifying it as a lipase inhibitor medication. The mechanism of action involves the inhibition of pancreatic lipase, which is an enzyme accountable for the hydrolysis of dietary triglycerides in the gastrointestinal tract. Xenical facilitates weight loss in overweight or obese individuals by inhibiting the absorption of fat.

The utilization of Xenical is recommended for the purpose of weight management in adult individuals whose body mass index (BMI) is equal to or greater than 30, or in those whose BMI is equal to or greater than 27 and who exhibit other risk factors such as hypertension, diabetes, or dyslipidemia. The intended use of this product is to be in combination with a diet that is reduced in calories and modifications to one's lifestyle.

Xenical should not be administered to individuals who have a documented hypersensitivity to Orlistat or any of its constituents. The utilization of this substance is contraindicated during gestation or lactation. The administration of Xenical is contraindicated in patients suffering from chronic malabsorption syndrome or cholestasis.

Xenical is presented in oral capsule dosage form. The active ingredient present in each capsule is Orlistat, with a concentration of 120 mg. The capsules are commonly characterized by a turquoise blue hue and bear the imprint "Xenical 120" on their exterior.

The prescribed dosing regimen for Xenical entails the administration of 120 mg of the medication orally thrice daily, coinciding with each primary meal. The optimal timing for the administration of Xenical is during or within an hour after the consumption of a meal that is rich in fat. In the event of a missed meal or a meal lacking in fat content, it is recommended to omit the administration of Xenical dosage. It is recommended that the daily consumption of fat, carbohydrates, and protein be evenly distributed across three primary meals.

In terms of administration considerations, it is imperative to adhere to a balanced and calorie-restricted diet that is abundant in fruits and vegetables while consuming Xenical. The recommended dietary intake suggests that the individual's daily caloric intake should consist of approximately 30% fat, with each primary meal comprising roughly 15 grams of fat. Distributing fat consumption uniformly over the course of the day is advised as a means of reducing the incidence of adverse gastrointestinal effects.

The duration of treatment with Xenical is typically established based on individualized considerations. The reduction in body weight is commonly observed during the initial fortnight of treatment, with the most significant outcome typically being witnessed within a span of six months. It is recommended to discontinue the use of Xenical if a patient fails to achieve a minimum of 5% reduction in their initial body weight after 12 weeks of treatment, as it may not be efficacious for that particular individual.

In the event of a missed or skipped dose of Xenical, it is recommended to omit the dose and instead take the next scheduled dose with the subsequent meal that contains fat. Overdose should be avoided. It is not advisable to compensate for a missed dose by administering a double dose. In the event of an overdose, the administration of a specific antidote is not currently available, and it is recommended to commence symptomatic treatment. In the event of severe symptoms, it is advisable to seek medical attention.

The adverse effects of Xenical primarily consist of gastrointestinal symptoms, including but not limited to oily spotting, flatus with discharge, fecal urgency, fatty or oily stools, and abdominal pain. These symptoms have been reported as the most frequently occurring adverse effects. The observed effects are typically of a mild nature and are attributed to the passage of unabsorbed fat through the gastrointestinal tract. Less frequently observed adverse reactions may comprise cephalalgia, urinary tract infections, and menstrual irregularities.

CHAPTER 5

POTENTIAL REACTIONS AND INTERACTIONS OF XENICAL

This response will provide a comprehensive analysis of the interactions and reactions associated with Xenical, including considerations such as drug interactions, adverse effects, contraindications, and precautionary measures.

The medication Xenical has the potential to decrease the blood concentrations of cyclosporine, which is a pharmaceutical agent utilized for immunosuppression. This interaction between the two drugs is classified as a drug interaction. It is imperative to conduct meticulous monitoring of cyclosporine levels when administering Xenical concurrently. Xenical has the potential to impede the anticoagulant properties of warfarin, a pharmacological agent utilized for blood thinning purposes. It is advisable to conduct routine surveillance of hemostatic indices.

Xenical has the potential to impact the absorption of levothyroxine, a pharmaceutical agent utilized for the purpose of thyroid hormone replacement therapy. The coadministration of Xenical with levothyroxine may necessitate a modification in the dosage of the latter. Xenical has the potential to reduce the serum concentrations of specific antiepileptic drugs, such as phenytoin and valproate. It is recommended to closely monitor the levels of therapeutic drugs.

Undesirable Effects: Xenical has the potential to induce various undesirable effects, albeit their manifestation may not be universal. Frequently encountered adverse reactions comprise:

The most commonly reported adverse reactions are related to the gastrointestinal (GI) system. These can manifest as oily spotting, fecal urgency, increased bowel movements, flatulence, and abdominal pain. The aforementioned effects are predominantly attributed to the undigested lipids traversing the gastrointestinal tract. Individuals may experience changes in stool consistency, such as fatty or oily stools, as a result of reduced absorption of dietary fat.

Xenical usage has been associated with infrequent occurrences of severe gastrointestinal bleeding, as reported in some cases.

Although uncommon, Xenical may elicit allergic reactions. Manifestations of an allergic reaction may encompass cutaneous eruptions, pruritus, edema, profound vertigo, or respiratory distress.

Hepatic impairment is a potential adverse effect that has been infrequently linked to the use of Xenical. Clinical manifestations of hepatic impairment encompass the discoloration of the integumentary system or sclerae (jaundice), acholic feces, dark urine, persistent emesis, abdominal discomfort, or unexplained exhaustion.

Xenical has contraindications in specific circumstances owing to possible hazards. The aforementioned items encompass: Individuals who have a documented hypersensitivity to orlistat or any of the constituents present in Xenical are advised against the use of this medication. Individuals with chronic malabsorption syndrome, a condition marked by inadequate nutrient absorption, are advised against the use of Xenical.

Individuals with cholestasis, a medical condition characterized by the obstruction of bile flow from the liver, are contraindicated for the use of Xenical.

The utilization of Xenical is not advised during pregnancy or lactation.

Precautions:

Individuals with specific medical conditions, such as type 2 diabetes, kidney stones, pancreatitis, or gallbladder disease, should exercise prudence when consuming Xenical due to the presence of coexisting conditions. It is recommended that individuals receive diligent supervision from a healthcare practitioner.

The administration of Xenical has been found to have a potential impact on the absorption of fat-soluble vitamins (namely, vitamins A, D, E, K) and beta-carotene when taken as a supplement. It may be imperative to supplement these vitamins to avert any potential deficiencies.

The optimal use of Xenical involves its combination with a low-fat diet that is also reduced in calorie content. Adhering to the prescribed dietary recommendations is crucial when consuming Xenical.

To summarize, Xenical is a pharmacological agent used to treat obesity by impeding the absorption of dietary lipids. Although it may prove efficacious for weight management purposes, it is crucial to exercise caution and remain cognizant of its potential interactions with other pharmaceuticals, potential adverse reactions, contraindications, and precautionary measures. It is advisable to seek the guidance of a healthcare practitioner prior to commencing any novel medication in order to ascertain its safety and suitability for use.

THE END

Made in the USA
Coppell, TX
22 April 2024

31609095R00024